HOW TO SHAPE UP YOUR HEALTH 2.0

"Enjoy good health."
—3 John 2

STAN TOLER

dustjacket

Dust Jacket Media Group
PO Box 721243
Oklahoma City, OK 73172
Info@DustJacket.com
Printed in the United States of America
ISBN: 978-1-947671-30-0

Writer: Stan Toler with Kevin Riggs

This Bible study is a companion book to Stan Toler's *Total Quality Life: Strategies for Purposeful Living*, expanded ed. (Indianapolis, Ind.: Wesleyan Publishing House, 2009).

This book contains advice and information related to health and medicine. It is not intended to replace medical advice and should be used to supplement rather than replace the regular care of a physician. Readers are encouraged to consult with their physicians regarding specific questions and concerns.

CONTENTS

WEEK 1

EAT WELL

RECOMMENDED READING

Total Quality Life, chapter 4, pages 53–58

Christians are disciples of Jesus Christ. The word *disciple* is related to the word *discipline*. You cannot be a disciple without being disciplined. I consider myself a fairly disciplined person. I am a self-starter and have never needed anyone looking over my shoulder to make sure I was doing what I was supposed to be doing. One area where many people struggle to remain disciplined once they reach adulthood, however, is with their health. For many in my generation, the first two decades were the most active years of our lives. As a result, we didn't concern ourselves much with our health and rarely worried about what or how much we ate. We didn't concern ourselves much with our weight, and we stayed in pretty good shape for the most part.

Once we reach adulthood, however, it is generally more difficult to stay active, and we have to start watching what we eat more carefully. Over the next six weeks, as we apply total quality life to our health, I want you to know we are all in the same boat. Maintaining physical fitness is a daily battle, and some days it is more of a struggle than others. When we experience victory in this battle, we achieve not only greater health, but greater satisfaction. Taking care of my health will make me a better husband, father, pastor, teacher, and friend; so I keep fighting.

To assist in obtaining better health, I am offering a health tip at the end of each day. Most of these tips are common sense. However, please note that these tips are in no way medical advice; they are simply suggestions. As always, check with your doctor before beginning anything new.

Total quality health starts with watching what we eat. We must eat well to live well.

DAY 1

DEUTERONOMY 14:1–21

Have you ever wondered about all those dietary restrictions God gave the Israelites back in the Old Testament? Why would he include such seemingly trivial things in his covenant with his people? What was the logic behind some animals being declared clean and others unclean?

Scholars usually offer one of four explanations for these dietary prohibitions. First, the restrictions might have been given for practical, hygienic reasons. In ancient times, some animals carried greater risks of diseases than others, so, following the dietary laws would probably have been better for a person's overall health. Another possible explanation is that these particular animals were declared off-limits because they were commonly associated with pagan worship and sacrifices. A third attempt to explain the prohibitions is that the clean and unclean animals were meant to symbolize good and evil. Finally, some think the lists may have been purely arbitrary on God's part, representing nothing more than God's desire that his children be different from the rest of society.

There is no way to know for sure which, if any, of these views is correct. The only hint of a reason the Bible gives is found in verse 21: "You are a people holy to the LORD your God." That statement is a summary of an earlier explanation about another restriction: "You are a people holy to the LORD your God. Out of all the peoples on the face of the earth, the LORD has chosen you to be his treasured possession" (v. 2). That explanation—that he was Israel's covenant God—was all God deemed necessary.

Many years later, Jesus declared all foods clean (Mark 7:19), and Peter had a vision that convinced him that the ancient dietary laws were no longer required by God (Acts 10:9–23). As a result, most Christians today don't follow these rules. Still, under God's new covenant, those who follow Jesus are God's "chosen people," and we are urged to live holy lives (1 Pet. 2:9–12). So, even though Christians are free from any specific rules or laws regarding our diet, we should not take this to mean that God is unconcerned about what or how we eat. Always remember and live by the words of the apostle Paul: "Whether you eat or drink or whatever you do, do it all for the glory of God" (1 Cor. 10:31).

DAILY HEALTH TIP

Add whole grain to your diet. The main benefit of a diet high in whole grain foods is a reduced risk of developing cardiovascular diseases. Examples of whole grain foods include: popcorn, brown rice, wild rice, oatmeal, and wheat.

QUESTIONS FOR REFLECTION

1. On a scale of one to ten (one being poor and ten being excellent), how would you rank your overall health? Why did you answer the way you did? What changes would you like to see in your life over the next six weeks?

2. What do you think of the four possible explanations given as to why God placed restrictions on the Israelites' diet? Which explanation do you think is the best? Why?

3. As a Christian, how should your attitude about dieting, eating, and being healthy, be different from a non-Christian?

PRAYER FOR TODAY

Lord, thank you for delivering me by your grace from the curse of the law and for choosing me to be your treasured possession. I want to glorify you in everything I do—even in what I eat and drink. Give me the resolve, focus, and discipline necessary to practice healthy eating habits. In the strong name of Jesus I pray. Amen.

DAY 2

GENESIS 3:1–19

On the sixth day of creation, God created humanity. He created man and woman in his image and likeness and said to them, "I give you every seed-bearing plant on the face of the whole earth and every tree that has fruit with seed in it. They will be yours for food. And to all the beasts of the earth and all the birds of the air and all the creatures that move on the ground—everything that has the breath of life in it—I give every green plant for food. And it was so" (Gen. 1:29–30). In the beginning, God said all food was good, but later he placed restrictions on what his people could eat, and today many of the things we eat could not be considered good food. So, what happened?

Sometime after creation—we are not told when or how long—Adam and Eve were enjoying a blissful existence in the garden, when a beautiful, crafty serpent convinced Eve to eat a certain piece of fruit that God had forbidden. The Hebrew word does not specify what kind of fruit; it is the more general term for any kind of fruit. So why do many people assume it was an apple? It all started in the fourth century when the Bible was translated into Latin. The serpent told Eve that once she ate the fruit, she would know "good and evil" (3:5). The Latin word for *evil* happens to be the same as the Latin word for *apple* (*malum*). As a result, people started associating the apple with the fruit Adam and Eve ate in the garden.

Because of the rebellion in the garden, God pronounced a judgment on the serpent (vv. 14–15), the woman (v. 16), the man (v. 17), and even creation itself. Of creation, God said, "Cursed is the ground because of you; through painful toil you will eat of it. . . . It will produce thorns and thistles for you. . . . By the sweat of your brow you will eat your food" (vv. 17–19).

Perhaps it was this part of the curse on creation that included the risks associated with certain types of food. What we can say for certain though, is that Adam and Eve's inability to overcome the temptations related to food is one that most of their descendants have wrestled with at one time or another. Sometimes this is because we eat to excess, rather than in moderation. Sometimes it is because we fill up on junk foods and highly processed foods rather than sticking with nature's nutrition. The good news is that God can give you both the desire and the power to resist temptation.

DAILY HEALTH TIP

Eat your vegetables, especially those that are fresh and in-season. Vegetables contain antioxidants that may help fight off certain cancers, as well as prevent heart disease and strokes. The well-worn guideline is still good advice: eat something green at every meal.

QUESTIONS FOR REFLECTION

1. What are some foods you eat that you know are bad for you? Why do you eat them?

2. Read Romans 8:19–21. What do you think Paul meant when he wrote, "Creation itself will be liberated from its bondage"? How do you think this applies to planting and harvesting?

3. How do you think God's redemption of our lives impacts our ability to live a healthy lifestyle?

PRAYER FOR TODAY

Father God, thank you for loving me unconditionally, for creating me in your image, and for providing for my redemption. Guide my every thought and action so that every choice I make—even in my food and drink—returns glory to you. In Jesus' wonderful name I pray. Amen.

DAY 3

PROVERBS 23:1–3, 19–21

The Bible gives plenty of room for us to enjoy the blessings of God's creation, including the delicious tastes of a skillfully prepared, nutritious meal. But the Bible also issues some strong warnings about overeating.

Near the end of the sixth century A.D., church leaders began to notice that most sins could be categorized under seven headings. Those seven headings became known as the seven deadly sins, and it was believed that all the evils in the world were rooted in these seven deadly sins: laziness (sloth), lust, anger, pride, envy, gluttony, and greed. Many church leaders have considered gluttony to be the deadliest of the deadly sins.

Proverbs warns us not to gorge ourselves on too much food, especially if we are an invited guest in someone's house. Proverbs also warns us to control our appetites because the person feeding us may be fattening us up for their own purposes (vv. 1–3). Gluttony is associated with excess in other areas, like drunkenness, and can lead a person to a life of poverty. However, the person who can control their appetite is considered wise (vv. 19–21).

Many are fortunate enough to live in an affluent society, but our abundance of food and drink has led in turn to an abundance of eating disorders—from obesity to bulimia to anorexia. We eat not just for daily sustenance or when we are hungry, but to hide our emotions, celebrate important events, close a business deal, or try and kill the pain of depression and loneliness. Those who are wise learn to say no, resist, and back away from the table, or, in the words of the writer of Proverbs, to "put a knife to [their] throat[s]" (v. 2) instead of to the meat. Don't take that verse literally; the writer was merely emphasizing the deceptive temptation to overindulge and the critical nature of controlling our appetites. In contrast, the way of wisdom is to learn to be satisfied with what our bodies need.

DAILY HEALTH TIP

Fruit makes a wonderful snack. Begin the practice of always having a bowl of fruit in your house. People who eat a lot of fruit are less likely to develop diabetes, Alzheimer's, and cancer. Fruit also provides your body with nutrients to fight off other infections, as well as to repair cells.

QUESTIONS FOR REFLECTION

1. How would you define gluttony? Why do you think church leaders considered gluttony to be the deadliest of sins? Do you agree with their assessment? Why or why not?

2. How do you think healthy eating habits can be an indication of one's desire to honor God?

PRAYER FOR TODAY

Heavenly Father, sanctify my life not only in word, but also in deed and behavior. Grant me the grace of self-control and help me to resist the temptation of overindulging in your good gifts. In the powerful name of Jesus. Amen.

DAY 4

DANIEL 1:1–21

Have you ever told a friend about a horrible dream you had the night before, and the first response from your friend was, "What did you eat last night?" We know instinctively that there is a relationship between what we eat and how well we sleep. We also know there is a relationship between what we eat and how much energy we have and how productive we are at work. Eating right makes a huge difference in our lives.

In the ancient world, when one nation conquered another, it was common for the victorious nation to claim the most gifted and talented young people from the conquered nation and educate them in the wisdom and customs of the conquering nation. This is precisely what happened to Daniel and his three friends Hananiah (Shadrach), Mishael (Meshach), and Azariah (Abednego) when the kingdom of Babylon went to war against the declining kingdom of Judah.

Daniel and his friends were deported to Babylon and suddenly found themselves in a privileged situation. They received specialized training and were provided food and drink from the king's table. "But Daniel resolved not to defile himself with the royal food and wine" (v. 8). It seems the royal diet did not square with the dietary guidelines in God's law, so Daniel refused to indulge in the sumptuous fare.

The official responsible for Daniel already thought well of him, so when Daniel requested a different diet for himself and his friends, the official granted the request. Their "special" diet consisted entirely of fresh vegetables and water. After ten days, the official noticed that

Daniel and his friends appeared healthier than those who were eating from the king's table, so he agreed to let them continue their diet. We can assume that Daniel and his friends were also more productive and energetic than the others because the official proceeded to put every one of the deported young men on Daniel's diet of vegetables and water.

Daniel was granted health and success because he was obedient to God even in matters of food and drink. God grant us the wisdom and courage to honor God in such things as well!

DAILY HEALTH TIP

Don't forget your protein, and lean protein is the best. Eat more fish, but not fried fish. Salmon and trout are excellent sources of protein. Don't skip breakfast either; eggs and milk are excellent sources of protein. Finally, skin your chicken before cooking and try to avoid processed meats.

QUESTIONS FOR REFLECTION

1. In what ways can the food you eat make a difference in how productive you are during your waking hours and the quality of sleep you get at night?

2. Can you think of ways in which you have "defiled" yourself by what you have eaten?

PRAYER FOR TODAY

Dear Lord, thank you for Daniel's example. Please help me to have a similar fortitude and resolve not to harm myself by what I eat. Instead, help me to follow a diet that will keep me healthy and productive in your kingdom. In Jesus' name. Amen.

DAY 5

JOHN 6:25–59

As important as it is to eat right, it is even more important to nourish your soul, and the only person who can truly nourish your soul is Jesus Christ. He is the "bread of life" (v. 35).

Many people followed Jesus not because of who he was, but of what he could do for them. Jesus said there were those who followed him "because [they] ate the loaves and had [their] fill" (v. 26). Previously, Jesus had fed five thousand men, women, and children with five loaves and two small fish (6:1–15). He then told the crowd, "Do not work for food that spoils, but for food that endures to eternal life" (v. 27). Who wouldn't want food that lasts for eternity, so the people said to Jesus, "Give us this bread" (v. 34). Jesus responded, "I am the bread of life. He who comes to me will never go hungry" (v. 35).

Jesus is the bread that never goes bad, never decays, and satisfies for all eternity.

In this passage, Jesus drew a simple comparison between himself and the manna God provided the Israelites in the wilderness: one is eternal and the other was temporary. Jesus said, "Your forefathers ate manna and died, but he who feeds on this bread will live forever" (v. 58). And just in case they misunderstood, Jesus spoke even more graphically: "I tell you the truth, unless you eat the flesh of the Son of Man and drink his blood, you have no life in you. Whoever eats my flesh and drinks my blood has eternal life. . . . For my flesh is real food and my blood is real drink. Whoever eats my flesh and drinks my blood remains in me, and I in him" (vv. 53–56). Pretty obvious isn't it? Unless you, by faith, participate with Jesus in his death, you do not have eternal life.

A person can eat all the right foods and be in perfect physical shape and still die. The benefits of a healthy diet are for this life and they are extremely important, but in order to live forever, a person must taste the Bread of Life, Jesus himself.

We have spent this week discussing the need to eat right and maintain a healthy balance. In no way do I mean for this last day to undermine anything that has already been said. It is extremely important to eat well so you can be more productive, happier, and healthier. And the habits that lead to health in this life are habits that will serve you well in God's kingdom. But physical health is worth little if you don't place your faith in Jesus Christ, asking him to feed your soul. Have you done so? Have you placed your faith in the Bread of Life?

DAILY HEALTH TIP

Make sure your diet is low in fat. As much as possible, avoid fats such as butter, saturated fats, animal fats, and dairy fats. Furthermore, avoid fast food restaurants. A low-fat diet is one of the primary keys to keeping your heart healthy.

QUESTIONS FOR REFLECTION

1. What do you think Jesus meant when he described himself as the "bread of life" (v. 35)? How would you explain what he meant to someone else?

2. "What good is it for a man to gain the whole world, yet forfeit his soul?" (Mark 8:36).

PRAYER FOR TODAY

Dear Jesus, thank you for offering yourself as the Bread of Life. Today and every day, I place my faith and trust in you. Sanctify my heart and life for your service by your love, mercy, and grace. In your name I pray. Amen.

WEEK 2

EXERCISE

RECOMMENDED READING

Total Quality Life, chapter 4, pages 60–61; chapter 8, pages 140–146

Exercise is important for everyone, but if your job requires more mental than physical work, exercise is a must. Something as simple as a brisk walk, or some other form of exercise, gets the blood flowing to your brain. Extra blood flow refreshes your mind. Exercise also releases chemicals (endorphins) into your blood stream. These chemicals give you a sense of satisfaction that positively affect your overall attitude and sense of well-being.

Total quality life involves taking care of your health, and a huge part of living a healthy lifestyle is exercise.

DAY 1

1 CORINTHIANS 9:24–27

The two greatest sporting events of New Testament times, the Olympic and Isthmian Games, both climaxed with a marathon race.

The Greek word translated *race* (v. 24) is *stadion*, the root for our English word *stadium*. Paul painted a word picture of marathon runners entering a stadium for the final leg of the great race. Paul said that all runners who compete in the marathon race endure a disciplined training regimen (v. 25).

You may never plan to run a marathon race, but staying in shape so you can live a total quality life still requires that you go through the agony of disciplining yourself, getting off the couch or out of bed to exercise.

But here is the thing to remember: While keeping in shape and exercising regularly is important for living a life of quality, even more important is keeping in shape spiritually. And the more you exercise physically the more energy you will have to exercise spiritually. Both physical and spiritual exercise go together.

DAILY HEALTH TIP

If you are going to start a new exercise program and you have not exercised in a significant amount of time, the most important tip is to start slowly. Gradually build up your speed, strength, and endurance. Starting too fast will set you up for failure.

QUESTIONS FOR REFLECTION

1. Approximately how much physical activity do you get each day at work? Is your job more physical or mental? What can you do this week to become more active?

2. How do you think physical exercise can benefit you, not only physically, but also spiritually? Have you ever considered the connection between physical exercise and spiritual growth?

PRAYER FOR TODAY

Heavenly Father, thank you for the gift of life in the body and for the ability to improve my physical health. As I exercise, please strengthen my body and consecrate it for use in your kingdom. In the name of Jesus I pray. Amen.

DAY 2

PHILIPPIANS 3:12–14

What does your exercise program look like? Did you exercise yesterday? What about today? One of the secrets to keeping an exercise program is accountability. Find someone who can exercise with you, or who can at least hold you accountable. Join an exercise group or a cycling class. In *Total Quality Life*, it says, "Accountability is a way to help us from straying too far from our objectives. Knowing we have to answer to someone for our actions can sometimes make the difference between a good and a bad choice" (p. 140).

Making yourself accountable to someone is what keeps you going when you would rather quit. The apostle Paul knew the importance of accountability, and he knew the importance of pressing on when the going got tough.

Paul's desire was to know Christ in a deep, personal way (Phil. 3:10–11). He knew he had not yet achieved that goal, but he was determined to keep going. He said, "I press on to take hold of that for which Christ Jesus took hold of me" (v. 12). When I see or hear the word *press*, I often think of a bench press or a leg press. When a person is working out with weights, trying to press heavier ones, they sometimes come to a near stop and then really exert themselves. What they are doing at that moment is "pressing into" the weight in order to get it to move. In the same way people push themselves to new limits physically, Paul said he did so to become like Jesus. Instead of turning away from Jesus when life gets difficult, press more into him.

Paul switched analogies from a person lifting weights to a sprinter, looking straight ahead and pushing his chest forward to cross the finish line. He wrote, "But one thing I do: Forgetting what is behind and straining toward what is ahead, I press on toward the goal to win the prize for which God has called me heavenward in Christ Jesus" (vv. 13–14).

Are you determined to get in shape and exercise so you can enjoy a higher quality of life? Are you as determined to strive and become like Jesus? I desperately want to be like Christ, but I know his work in me is not done, so I press on and keep running. What about you?

DAILY HEALTH TIP

A good way to exercise regularly is to get into a routine so it becomes a part of your life. Exercise at the same time of the day. Work out a schedule for what you are going to do on Monday, Wednesday, and Friday, and another schedule for Tuesday, Thursday, and Saturday.

QUESTIONS FOR REFLECTION

1. Have you started an exercise program in the past only to stop after a few times? Why did you stop? What can you do differently this time to keep on keeping on?

2. Who can you make yourself accountable to for your exercise program?

PRAYER FOR TODAY

Father, thank you for creating the human body to move, walk, and run. Guide me to find the right accountability partner to help me in my journey to better health—both physically and spiritually. In Jesus' name I pray. Amen.

DAY 3

HEBREWS 12:1–13

o pain, no gain!

A friend once severely twisted his ankle playing basketball. He didn't get it X-rayed right away, and he spent a couple of days limping around. Since he couldn't put all his weight on his ankle, he walked around on his tip-toes. When he finally went and had it X-rayed, his doctor put him on crutches for three weeks. The doctor's advice was that if he couldn't walk correctly ("heel toe, heel toe," he said), my friend should not walk at all. When recovering from an injury, "no pain, no gain" is bad advice, and it could make matters worse. However, when it comes to pushing yourself beyond what you thought were your limits, no pain, no gain can be good advice.

The writer of Hebrews encourages us to keep running because there are people who have gone on before us in the grandstands cheering us on, as if we were near the finish line of a marathon. The writer says we should be motivated by their faithful examples, and we should get rid of everything that slows us down so we can "run with perseverance the race marked out for us" (v. 1). Then the writer gives us the no-pain-no-gain principle by stating, "Endure hardship as discipline. . . . No discipline seems pleasant at the time, but painful. Later on, however, it produces a harvest of righteousness and peace for those who have been trained by it" (vv. 7, 11).

Physically, as you begin to exercise, you will go through a period of time where your body rebels. Every muscle will hurt; spasm may even occur. Every joint in your body will scream. But in the long run, your body will be stronger. So fight through the fatigue and soreness. The reward is better health.

Likewise, spiritually you may go through difficult times. You may find out the more committed to Christ you become, the more difficult life becomes. But hang in there; your spiritual muscles are being developed and you will be stronger than you ever thought possible.

DAILY HEALTH TIP

Look for opportunities to be more active during the course of your workday. Take the stairs instead of the elevator. Park in the back of the parking lot and walk. Go to the mall during your lunch break and walk. Stand up and stretch for a few minutes every hour. There are plenty of opportunities to be active during the day if you will take advantage of them.

QUESTIONS FOR REFLECTION

1. Who are some faithful believers you have known who have died and are now numbered with the "cloud of witnesses," cheering you on? Are you running a race for which they can be proud?

2. Can you think of a difficult time you went through spiritually that now, looking back, you know made you stronger? Can you think of a physical injury you had that took daring determination to overcome? How can you apply that same determination to your spiritual life?

PRAYER FOR TODAY

Lord God, thank you for all the examples you have given me of people who have run a good spiritual race. Thank you for the difficult times that have developed my spiritual strength. I pray you will take the physical pain I am experiencing right now and use it to make me stronger. Thank you for loving me and caring about every detail of my life. In the strong name of Jesus I pray. Amen.

DAY 4

ISAIAH 40:25–31

People who often engage in running, swimming, biking, or other activities for long distances describe an interesting phenomenon known as the "second wind." After they exerted a certain amount of energy and effort, they would go through a time where continuing seemed nearly impossible, and they would begin to think they would not be able to finish. But then, as they fought that feeling and pressed, something amazing would happen: they would get their second wind and find the strength to complete the miles, laps, or whatever.

What is a second wind? It's not a scientific term, but a second wind occurs when you are exerting yourself mentally or physically. You reach a point of exhaustion, and everything within you is saying, "Stop! Quit! You can't go any further!" But as you refuse to quit, and keep pushing yourself, something unexpected occurs. Your body quits aching, you get more energy, and almost effortlessly (sometimes robotically), you keep going, no longer feeling the pain and fatigue.

When we become spiritually fatigued and are ready to quit, the prophet Isaiah tells us where our second wind originates.

In Isaiah 40, God comforted his people, letting them know that their time of trial was almost over. He encouraged them to trust in his sovereignty—"To whom will you compare me?" (v. 25)—and to rely on his strength. The prophet says, God "will not grow tired or weary, and his understanding no one can fathom" (v. 28).

It is precisely because of God's sovereignty, strength, and wisdom that he can be trusted, and when we trust him instead of ourselves, he gives us his strength. He gives us our second wind so we can continue (vv. 30–31). When we place our hope in him, he renews our strength, enabling us to soar like eagles and run and walk without getting tired (v. 31).

I love the picture the prophet paints of an eagle in flight. The eagle, with its beauty, majesty, grace, and power, harnessing the wind and soaring at great speed without flapping its wings, is something to behold. God is telling us to quit flapping our own wings, and to soar on the power he has provided.

DAILY HEALTH TIP

One way to stay consistent with your exercise program is to use variety. Variety is the spice of life and will keep things from getting monotonous. Swim one day, walk the next, jog the next, lift weights the next, go on a bike ride the next, and so on and so forth.

QUESTIONS FOR REFLECTION

1. In what ways can relying on God's wisdom and strength make your life easier?

2. What do you think it means to say that God will renew our strength and enable us to "soar on wings like eagles" (v. 31)?

PRAYER FOR TODAY

Father God, teach me to soar with you, relying on your wisdom and strength, instead of relying on my own resources. Forgive me for when I choose to do things my own way. As I press on, I trust in you to renew my strength and enable me to soar like an eagle. In the mighty name of Jesus I pray. Amen.

DAY 5

PROVERBS 4:18–27

Running is one of the simplest yet most challenging forms of exercise. You can run nearly anywhere—on pavement, gravel, grass, or dirt. Or you can run in place or on a treadmill in the privacy of your own home. Running requires a minimum of equipment: comfortable clothes and a suitable pair of shoes. If you like running, more power to you. But running is also a demanding discipline—physically and mentally—and can result in unexpected aches and even injuries. When you run, you have to watch your steps carefully and make sure the path you are running is passable.

Many people who run or do other exercise outside prefer to do so in the morning before daylight so they can witness that "first gleam of dawn" (v. 18). There is something life affirming about the beginning of a new day. Each new day offers hope, and the writer of Proverbs said that is what the path of the righteous is like. Running at night can be tricky. There are things along the way that could make you stumble, things you will never see until it is too late; and that is what the "way of the wicked" is like (v. 19).

One great thing about running is that it gets your heartbeat going. Running is great cardiovascular exercise, and we all know the heart is the most important muscle. Likewise, spiritually, the greatest cardiovascular exercise we can do is to listen to the wisdom found in God's Word, apply it to our lives, and obey it. The writer of Proverbs tells us to keep words of wisdom within our hearts (v. 21), "for they are life to those who find them and health to a man's whole body" (v. 22). Physically and spiritually, there is nothing more important than taking care of your heart, "for it is the wellspring of life" (v. 23).

All week long, our focus has been on the importance of exercising to remain in good health. Along the way, an attempt has been made to point out a connection between physical exercise and spiritual growth. The better our health is, physically, the better we can serve God by serving others. Letting our physical health decline not only harms us physically, but it also takes its toll spiritually. The purpose for making this connection is to motivate us to see that physical exercise is a must so we can be all God wants us to be. Physical exercise is a necessity if we desire to live a life of total quality.

DAILY HEALTH TIP

Drink lots of water. Drink a cup of water before, during, and after your work out. Also, it is best not to exercise right after meals, or when it is extremely hot or humid.

QUESTIONS FOR REFLECTION

1. What do you think it means to describe the path of the righteous as "the first gleam of dawn" (v. 18)? How would you describe that analogy to someone else?

2. How would you explain the connection between physical exercise and spiritual growth? What does that connection mean to you?

PRAYER FOR TODAY

Lord, thank you for this week and the emphasis on exercise, both physical and spiritual exercise. I trust your saving and sanctifying work in my heart. Help me to take care of my physical body so that I can be the best I can be for you. I pray in the name of your Son Jesus. Amen.

WEEK 3

REST

RECOMMENDED READING

Total Quality Life, chapter 4, pages 58–59; chapter 8, pages 121–125

Imagine being part of a family whose members have been slaves—working continuously, without a day off, break, or vacation—for the last four hundred years. Imagine working all those years yourself without a break, and then, suddenly, you are set free. The only condition of your freedom is to leave the country where you've been enslaved and begin a long journey across a hot desert. Before, you lived in a state of bondage, but now, each day is a fight for survival. Each day, you journey in the hot sun and search for a single day's worth of food and water for you and your family. One day, a man stands before the entire clan, claiming he has heard from God. The man tells you, among other things, that God has said you are to rest on the last day of the week. You are not to work or even gather food and water.

Is he insane? You and your family are barely surviving on what you gather day-to-day. How can you take an entire day off to do nothing but rest?

Total quality life requires total quality health, and an important component of good health is getting adequate rest.

DAY 1

Exodus 20:1–17

Many believers will tell you that in today's culture, keeping a weekly Sabbath is not practical, and since we are now under grace and not under the law, there is no reason to even try to keep the Sabbath. Even though we are under grace, we still need adequate rest.

The fourth commandment (vv. 8–11) is the longest commandment and includes the most explanation.

The word *Sabbath* means "to rest from labor." The basis for taking a weekly day to rest is the example of God during creation week, when God worked six days then rested on the seventh. The word *holy* means to "set apart as consecrated." The Sabbath command is to take one day in seven and separate that day to God by resting your body and renewing your soul. You were not made to keep going and going and going. Your body needs time to recover, and you need a reminder that all you have is from God. Your total dependence is on him. If the Israelites, who were in a life-and-death struggle for survival, could take a day off each week to rest, relax, reflect, and reenergize, then so can you. Your body needs it; your soul needs it; and God commands it.

DAILY HEALTH TIP

If you usually wake up tired, you may have some type of sleep disorder. Schedule an appointment with your doctor to discuss the possibility of a sleep study. Check with your insurance to see if it will pay for such a study.

QUESTIONS FOR REFLECTION

1. When was the last time you took a day off to relax and rejuvenate your body and soul? What excuses have you made for not taking a day off? When was the last time you went on a vacation?

2. For most Christians, Sunday has become the Sabbath. But Sundays have also become one of the busiest days of the week. What can you do this Sunday to truly rest and reflect on the goodness of God?

PRAYER FOR TODAY

Heavenly Father, help me to keep the principle of the Sabbath without becoming legalistic. Teach me to see that a day of rest is needed, not only for my body, but also for my soul. In Jesus' name I pray. Amen.

DAY 2

MARK 2:23–28

Part of yesterday's prayer was, "Help me to keep the principle of the Sabbath without becoming legalistic." This can be a difficult thing to do.

The original Sabbath commandment prohibited any type of physical labor. Later Jewish scholars defined and redefined the definition of physical labor. In other words, they forgot the principle of a day of rest and made it into a matter of keeping the law. Jesus violated their legalism. Here is what happened.

Jesus and his disciples, on a Sabbath day, were walking through a grain field (the walking violated the rule), and as they walked, they pulled the heads of grain off with their hands, rubbed their hands together to separate the husks from the kernels, blew the lighter husks away, and then ate the kernels. The Pharisees considered what they did physical labor, so they condemned them for violating the fourth commandment.

You might be thinking, wouldn't they also be guilty of stealing the grain? The answer is no. Under the Mosaic law, landowners were required to leave some grain for travelers to pick (see Deut. 23:25). What Jesus and his disciples did was permissible, but the Pharisees objected because they did it on the Sabbath. Separating the husks from the kernels was considered threshing, and blowing the husks away was considered winnowing. Both, according to the Pharisees' tradition, violated the Sabbath law.

Jesus reminded them that David had done something similar (see 1 Sam. 21:1–9), and then he identified the principle behind the law by saying, "The Sabbath was made for man, not man for the Sabbath" (Mark 2:27). In other words, God established the Sabbath principle of rest for the benefit of people, not to put them in bondage to rules and regulations. God did not need to take a day off at the end of creation week because he was tired. He took a day off to show us how important rest is to our overall health.

Did you know you can live longer without food and water than you can without sleep? That should tell us the importance of rest. There is nothing spiritual about working days and weeks without a break. In fact, doing so could be considered immoral. The Sabbath principle teaches us to trust God every day and follow his example because he knows what is best for us. Observing a day of rest and renewal reminds us of our total dependence on God.

DAILY HEALTH TIP

Most adults need between seven and nine hours of sleep every night to maintain optimum health. A lack of adequate sleep could lead to health problems like obesity, high blood pressure, diabetes, and premature aging. So, make sure you're getting enough sleep.

QUESTIONS FOR REFLECTION

1. How do you think you can keep the principle of a consistent Sabbath rest without becoming legalistic? Why should you even try?

2. How much sleep do you average each night? Is that enough? What can you do to get more rest?

3. Do you agree with the statement that working days and weeks without a break could be considered immoral? Why or why not?

PRAYER FOR TODAY

Creator God, thank you for caring so much for humanity that you built rest into our systems. Help me to achieve high-quality rest so I can be more productive for you and my family. I pray this in Jesus' name. Amen.

DAY 3

MATTHEW 11:25–30

Have you ever had the experience of trying to solve a problem, work with your hands, or finish a project, and you just can't seem to get it right? And the more you try, the more mistakes you make? The best thing you can do in that situation is to stop, rest, and get back to it later. It's amazing how things can look different and even easier after a good night's sleep.

When we push ourselves harder and become fatigued, small problems become big, and minor issues become major. Sometimes the best thing you can do physically, emotionally, and spiritually, is to take a nap. The importance of rest cannot be overstated. In today's Scripture reading, we learn where real rest comes from.

When my boys were babies, I loved to watch them sleep. A sleeping baby is the epitome of rest and peace. As an adult, don't you wish you could rest like a child? Jesus reminds us of the importance of childlike faith in coming to God (vv. 25–26). He also reminds us that the only way to know God is by knowing him (v. 27).

Then Jesus issued an incredible invitation. He said (and still says today), "Come to me, all you who are weary and burdened, and I will give you rest" (v. 28). To be weary means to be tired from hard work. To be burdened means to be loaded down with a heavy weight. Work can be tiresome and life can be burdensome. Do you ever feel overworked, overwhelmed, and overstressed?

What you need is rest, and that is what Jesus invites you to have. But it's not only physical rest he wants to give you, but spiritual rest as well.

Jesus says that in him "you will find rest for your souls" (v. 29). Nothing can refresh the mind, body, and spirit like rest. Jesus did not come to add to the pressures of life. He came to redeem us from the pressures of life and give us rest. The rest Jesus gives keeps us safe in the middle of storms, calm in the middle of difficulties, and at peace in the middle of chaos.

DAILY HEALTH TIP

One very important aspect of mental health is learning to do nothing, allowing the mind time to idle and recharge. Learning to be idle allows you to gather your thoughts, gain perspective, and relieve stress. The Bible says, "Be still, and know that I am God" (Ps. 46:10).

QUESTIONS FOR REFLECTION

1. How would you describe the rest and peace of a sleeping baby? Do you think that type of rest and peace is possible as an adult? Why or why not?

2. How would you describe the spiritual rest that we can have in Christ Jesus to someone else?

PRAYER FOR TODAY

Dear Jesus, I very much want the rest that you offer. Right now, I come to you in childlike faith. I place my complete trust in you. O Lord, I pray for rest so my strength can be renewed. Thank you for loving me and for giving me both physical and spiritual rest. In your holy name. Amen.

DAY 4

PSALM 37:1–11

By commanding us to rest, God is not advocating laziness. Quite the contrary. We were created to work and be active. But God knows we are most productive when we are rested. Life is not a sprint, but a marathon. You have to rest; you have to take a break if you desire to run the marathon of life effectively and efficiently.

It is easy to be envious of other people's success. At times, that envy motivates us to work harder and longer hours. During those times, we might be tempted to skip breakfast or lunch or to work weekends. "It's only temporary," we tell ourselves. "I'm just trying to get ahead." We work hard to keep up with the Joneses, and we don't understand why the Joneses are so successful when they are not living a godly life, while we struggle trying to do what is right.

David, the composer of Psalm 37, tells us not to be envious of such people because one day they will wither and die (vv. 1–2). Instead, we should "trust in the LORD and do good" (v. 3). It is never wrong to do right, and it is never a waste of time to do good.

If you will trust in God and delight in him, "he will give you the desires of your heart" (v. 4). And, as if that promise isn't enough, God promises to "make your righteousness shine like the dawn, the justice of your cause like the noonday sun" (v. 6). One day, God will set the record straight. One day, God will make things right. Meanwhile, rest in God's wisdom and power. "Be still before the LORD and wait patiently for him" (v. 7). When the time is right, "the meek will inherit the land and enjoy great peace" (v. 11).

So, don't worry yourself sick, and don't get your life out of balance trying to keep up with other people. Live the life God gave you, enjoying his presence and committing your all to him. In the end, you will not be sorry. In the end, God will give you what you most desire because what you most desire will be what he wants for you.

What a wonderful promise!

DAILY HEALTH TIP

Learn to take a power nap. A power nap lasts no longer than ten to twenty minutes and has proven to increase alertness and productivity during the workday. Longer naps can cause sustained drowsiness, but a short power nap in the middle of your day can provide a fresh burst of new ideas and energy.

QUESTIONS FOR REFLECTION

1. Have you ever been envious of people who are not following Jesus? What was the reason for your envy? How did you deal with it? Why is it so emotionally, physically, and spiritually draining to be envious of others?

2. What do you think it means to say, "The meek will inherit the land and enjoy great peace" (v. 11)?

PRAYER FOR TODAY

Heavenly Father, thank you for your love. I consecrate my life and my plans to you. No longer will I strive to keep up with other people. With your help, I will strive only to live for you, knowing that you know what is best. In the mighty name of Jesus I pray. Amen.

DAY 5

HEBREWS 4:1–11

This week we have been discussing the importance of adequate rest in maintaining optimal health. God has commanded that we rest. When we don't rest, we abuse our bodies and do harm to ourselves physically, emotionally, and spiritually. Today's passage teaches us that, ultimately, followers of Jesus Christ have been promised an eternal rest.

When I was learning to teach the Bible, I was taught that when you see the word *therefore* in the Bible, you should ask yourself, "What's the *therefore* there for?" The *therefore* of Hebrews 4:1 ties what the writer is about to say to what has been said in the previous chapter. Near the end of Hebrews 3, the writer discussed the Israelites and their failure to believe in the promise of God that they would enter the Promised Land, a land of rest. Now, today, God is still promising that we can enter his rest. Therefore, we should not be like the Israelites, who did not enter God's rest because of their unbelief. "For we also have had the gospel preached to us, just as they did; but the message they heard was of no value to them, because those who heard did not combine it with faith. Now we who have believed enter that rest" (vv. 2–3). Place your faith in Jesus Christ.

Are you entering the rest that God has promised? Are you tired of doing things your own way? Are you exhausted from carrying your own burdens? Are you fatigued by worrying about things you cannot control? Are you ready to take a break? Are you ready to rest?

In Jesus Christ, there is hope, peace, and rest. When you come to God and repent of your sins and place your faith in Jesus, you are promised eternal life. In addition, you are promised abundant life here on earth (see John 10:10).

"There remains, then, a Sabbath-rest for the people of God; for anyone who enters God's rest also rests from his own work, just as God did from his. Let us, therefore, make every effort to enter that rest" (Heb. 4:9–11).

DAILY HEALTH TIP

One of the single most important things you can do for your overall health and well-being is to learn to relax. When you relax, your body has an opportunity to unwind. Relaxing also slows your heart rate, reduces blood pressure, and increases blood flow to your muscles.

QUESTIONS FOR REFLECTION

1. What do you think it means to enter God's rest? Have you done so?

2. How can entering God's rest provide not only rest in eternity, but rest in this present life as well?

PRAYER FOR TODAY

Lord, sanctify my life by your love, mercy, and grace, so that I may enter into your rest. In the name of Jesus I pray. Amen.

WEEK 4

REDUCE STRESS

RECOMMENDED READING

Total Quality Life, chapter 4, pages 61–62

Everyone has stress in their lives, but not all stress is bad. Feelings of stress are a natural reaction to the pressures and demands we face in life. Stress is one of our body's defense responses. Stress can serve to give us the extra energy and strength we need to accomplish a specific task. This type of positive stress, called eustress, is usually short-lived and can help you emotionally, mentally, and physically. However, most of the time when we talk about stress, we talk about the negative type of stress, known as distress. Distress can lead to anxiety, depression, ulcers, and a host of other physical problems. Distress can start immediately or can result from prolonged periods of eustress without allowing our bodies a chance to recover.

I am convinced most of the stress in our lives is self-imposed distress. We are overly stressed because of the lifestyles we have chosen to live. We are stressed because we have forgotten what is really important and because our lives are out of balance.

If you and I are going to live a healthy, total quality life, then we must learn how to deal with stress.

DAY 1

PSALM 27

Mark Twain once commented, "I have been through some terrible things in my life, some of which actually happened." Many people live in unfounded fear. Living that way can be extremely stressful. In Psalm 27, David put these unfounded fears into perspective. Since God is our light, our salvation, and our defender, we have nothing to fear and no reason to be afraid. Regardless of what we are facing—real or imagined—we can be confident that God is our protector, he hears our voice and will never leave or forsake us.

Whatever it is you are facing in life—whether pressures at home, work, church, or health—there is no need to be afraid. God may not immediately deliver you from your troubles, but he will walk with you through them. God is your stronghold, so "be strong and take heart and wait for the LORD" (v. 14).

DAILY HEALTH TIP

Stress—eustress or distress—can cause health problems or make health problems worse. If you feel some of your physical symptoms are caused by stress, make an appointment and talk about it with your doctor. It is important to make sure these symptoms are not caused by other health problems.

QUESTIONS FOR REFLECTION

1. How would you explain the difference between eustress and distress to someone else? Can you think of examples when you experienced good stress? Can you think of examples when you experienced bad stress?

2. What do you think it means to say God is your stronghold?

PRAYER FOR TODAY

Father God, life is so full of stress. At times, I feel pressure from so many different angles. Lord, I look to you for strength and help. I trust in you as my stronghold. I praise you for what you have done and what you will do. In Jesus' name I pray. Amen.

DAY 2

MATTHEW 6:25–34

Worry and stress often go together; worrying causes stress, and stress leads to worrying. People who worry a lot are usually less happy, and they tend to make those around them less happy too. In today's Scripture reading, Jesus speaks to our worry.

In the middle of Jesus' famous Sermon on the Mount, he said, "Therefore I tell you, do not worry" (v. 25). He told his disciples not to worry about their lives, bodies, clothes, food, or homes (vv. 25–31). He said that worrying about these things is what pagans do, not people who trust in God (v. 32). Jesus said, "Therefore do not worry about tomorrow, for tomorrow will worry about itself. Each day has enough trouble of its own" (v. 34).

Think of all the emotional energy we spend worrying about things we cannot control. Worrying about something does absolutely nothing to help or change the situation. After all, "Who of you by worrying can add a single hour to his life?" (v. 27).

Living a total quality life requires that we stop worrying and learn to trust God by seeking "first his kingdom and his righteousness" (v. 33). As we learn to do that, God promises he will take care of all the details about our lives that have caused us to worry.

DAILY HEALTH TIP

If you feel overwhelmed, prioritize. Do what you can do, and leave it all in God's hands. Address the problems you can solve, and don't worry about things you cannot control.

QUESTIONS FOR REFLECTION

1. Do you think worry is compatible with faith? Why or why not?

2. What do you think Jesus meant when he told us not to worry about tomorrow because "each day has enough trouble of its own" (v. 34)? Is this good news or bad news?

PRAYER FOR TODAY

Heavenly Father, I don't want my life to be wasted by fretting and worrying over things that are beyond my control. I give you all my worries and concerns, and I pray for your will to be done in my life. In the powerful name of Jesus I pray. Amen.

DAY 3

1 PETER 5:6–11

An important first step in dealing with stress in your life is learning to recognize when you are feeling stressed. Some physical signs your body is under stress include tension in your shoulders and neck or clenching your hands into fists. When you sense your body responding to stress, it is time to take action to reduce that stress. Read the Bible, start praying daily, and seek to grow in God's grace. For some people, listening to Christian music helps reduce stress and release the tension in their muscles.

The apostle Peter wrote to give encouragement to a group of believers who were going through difficult times and tremendous stress. At the end of his beautiful letter, Peter told us the best way to deal with stress: "Cast all your anxiety on him because he cares for you" (v. 7). Let that promise sink in. To cast means to throw, and we are not told to throw some of our stress and anxiety on Jesus or just the really big stuff, but to throw all of our anxiety on him. Peter is using a play on words here. Other words for anxiety are *concern* or *worry*. Peter is saying, "Throw all your concerns on him because he is concerned for you." What a great promise!

What are you anxious about? What makes you concerned and worried? What keeps you up at night and causes that pain in your back or gives you a headache? The only solution is to take your anxiety and throw it to Jesus. Let your problems become his problems. He cares deeply for you and his shoulders are more than broad enough to carry you and what troubles you.

What happens when you transfer your anxiety to Jesus? The God who saved you by his grace and promises you eternal life will "restore you and make you strong, firm and steadfast. To him be the power for ever and ever. Amen" (vv. 10–11).

DAILY HEALTH TIP

Exercise is an excellent way to deal with stress. Exercise helps you relieve tension and releases chemicals into your brain that make you feel better. Exercise also helps you stay in shape and maintain better overall health.

QUESTIONS FOR REFLECTION

1. What are some physical signs that let you know when you are under a great deal of stress? What do you do when you first see those signs?

2. What are some things you can do as an outward expression of casting your anxieties on God? How would you explain what that means to someone else?

PRAYER FOR TODAY

Lord, through faith I am throwing all of my cares, concerns, and worries to you. I am asking you to relieve me of the stress I am under. Teach me how to deal with the stress in my life. Show me the changes I need to make and the things that I can do to reduce stress. Thank you for caring for me. In the majestic name of Jesus I pray. Amen.

DAY 4

PSALM 46

What do you fear? Whatever it is, there is probably a name for that fear. For example, do you fear failure? If so, you have a condition known as atychiphobia. Do you hate to read? If you do, you might have bibliophobia. Are you afraid of peanut butter getting stuck to the roof of your mouth? If so, then you suffer from arachibutyrophobia. And if you are afraid of fear itself, then you have phobophobia.

The psalmist says that even in the middle of your present trouble and even if the whole earth should collapse, there is still no reason to fear because God is "our refuge and strength" (v. 1).

Even in a time of war, natural disasters, and man-made calamities, God is still our fortress. He speaks and "the earth melts" (v. 6) and "wars cease to the ends of the earth" (v. 9). God is in control when things are going well, and he is in control when things are chaotic.

Instead of living in fear, our response should be to "be still, and know that [he is] God" (v. 10). The Hebrew word translated "be still" could also be translated "relax." There is no need to be afraid; there is no need to be stressed. Take a deep breath, relax, and then you will know that God is God, and he is still in control.

A friend who likes scuba diving once told me that if you get tangled in fishing line or some other obstruction while diving, your natural instinct is to try to fight your way out. But the more you try to fight the entanglement, the more entangled you become. The best thing to do is to relax, stop moving, and be still. Once you have done that, you can calmly get yourself out of the situation.

We live our lives at a hectic pace and rarely take time to relax. When faced with difficulties, we immediately try to fight our way out. But often, all the fighting makes the situation worse. We need to stop, be quiet, and wait until we hear from God. Then we can get ourselves out of the tangles and snares and move forward. When faced with difficulties, trials, and tribulations, we can either be stressed or get still.

DAILY HEALTH TIP

Train your body to relax. Start with one muscle. Hold it tight for a few seconds and then relax. Start with the muscles in your feet and work your way up through the rest of your body. Stretch and get going!

QUESTIONS FOR REFLECTION

1. What are your deepest fears? (If you say you have no fears, maybe you have a fear of being vulnerable. Everyone has fears.) What do you do to control those fears?

2. What can you do this week to relax and be still so you can hear from God? What changes do you need to make to your schedule to allow time to relax and be still?

PRAYER FOR TODAY

Father, thank you for being my refuge and strength. Thank you for always being in control, even when things seem out of control. I pray that you will teach me to relax and be still in the midst of difficulties so I can hear from you. In the peaceful name of Jesus I pray. Amen.

DAY 5

JOHN 14:15–27

Jesus' disciples were getting a little stressed because they were not sure what was going to happen next. Jesus had been telling them he was leaving and that they were not to be troubled because he would return for them. But the disciples didn't feel ready for him to go. Jesus comforted them by telling them that when he left he would not leave them alone. Rather, he would send someone to comfort, teach, and walk with them—a Counselor.

The Greek word translated "Counselor" is *parakletos*, which means "one called alongside another." This Counselor is the Holy Spirit. As a follower of Jesus Christ, I have no reason to fear because the Holy Spirit, the third person of the Trinity, is always with me. The Holy Spirit is more than a conscience, or a still small voice telling me right from wrong. He is much better than a spirit guide or mantra. The Holy Spirit is God himself—a real person who wants a personal relationship with me.

Jesus described the Holy Spirit as "another Counselor" (v. 16). What he meant was that the Holy Spirit would be another of the same kind, not another of a different kind. In other words, Jesus was promising another Counselor, just like himself. The implication is that the Holy Spirit is to you and me what Jesus was to his disciples. What an awesome thought! Through the Holy Spirit, we have access to the same person, power, and potential the disciples had through Jesus Christ. The way the Holy Spirit will be to us what Jesus was to the disciples is by teaching us and reminding us of everything Jesus has taught (v. 26). "Peace

I leave with you; my peace I give you. . . . Do not let your hearts be troubled and do not be afraid" (v. 27).

We can be overwhelmed by stress when we try to do things and handle difficulties by ourselves. Jesus did not want us to live life that way. The Holy Spirit is there to walk beside us and to take the stress from our lives by guiding us and reminding us of the promises of God.

DAILY HEALTH TIP

Develop a hobby. Find something you enjoy doing that is totally unrelated to what you do for a living. Developing such a hobby will get your mind off your circumstances, challenge your mind, and prove to be a valuable source of stress relief.

QUESTIONS FOR REFLECTION

1. What do you think it means to say that the Holy Spirit has been called to come alongside you? Do you find that truth comforting? How, and in what way?

2. What do you think it means to say that the Holy Spirit is to you and me what Jesus was to the disciples? How would living out that truth reduce stress in your life?

PRAYER FOR TODAY

Dear Father, thank you for your Son who died for me, and thank you for your Holy Spirit who is with me now, walking alongside me, guiding me in your truth. Sanctify me by your Spirit to walk in your truth and rest in your power. In Jesus' name I pray. Amen.

WEEK 5

AVOID HARMFUL SUBTANCES AND BEHAVIORS

RECOMMENDED READING

Total Quality Life, chapter 4, page 63; chapter 7, pages 111–113

Total quality health involves avoiding harmful substances and behaviors. Some harmful substances and behaviors are obvious—like illegal drugs or abuse of alcohol. Others are not as obvious—like nicotine, fatty foods, abuse of prescription drugs, and a host of other things. As we go through this week, every day's Scripture reading will come from the apostle Paul.

DAY 1

ROMANS 6:1–14

We are no longer under the law but grace, and I am so thankful for that fact. However, not being under the law is not a license to do whatever we feel like doing. Grace frees us, not so we can break the law, but so we can be free from the bondage of the law and sin to live a life that is holy and pleasing to God.

The purpose of the laws in the Old Testament was to show us how perfect and holy God is, how sinful we really are, and our need for a Savior. Before grace, we did not have the power to be free from sin. We were slaves to our natural desires. In our degenerate state, our bodies were instruments of wickedness (v. 13).

But now, because of the grace of God in Jesus Christ, we have died to sin and have been set free. Our bodies are no longer to be abused because now we belong to God as "instruments of righteousness" (v. 13). "For sin shall not be your master, because you are not under law, but under grace" (v. 14).

Do you see the application to your health and the importance of avoiding harmful substances? What you place in your body is a sign of whose instrument you are. Another word for *instrument* is *tool*. Your body is either a tool used for destruction or a tool in the hands of the Master Carpenter. Don't abuse God's instrument—your body—by feeding it unhealthy substances or by allowing it to rust, corrode, or breakdown for lack of care.

DAILY HEALTH TIP

I know it sounds cliché, but the first step to overcoming any type of addiction is admitting you have an addiction. Once you admit that some substance or activity has control of you, it is easier to get control back. Remember, however, as a follower of Jesus Christ, self-control is ultimately Holy Spirit control. Admit you have a problem and you need Holy Spirit power to conquer that problem.

QUESTIONS FOR REFLECTION

1. How do you think recognizing you are under grace and not under law should motivate you to live a holy life?

2. What steps can you take, this week, to ensure your body is used as a tool for righteousness and not a tool for wickedness?

PRAYER FOR TODAY

Dear God, teach me what it means to have died to sin and been brought back to life in Christ. Cleanse me and set me apart to live a Spirit-controlled life. Forgive me for how I have abused my body in the past. Today, I offer myself to you as an instrument of righteousness. In the strong name of Jesus. Amen.

DAY 2

ROMANS 6:15–23

Did you know there are more people in slavery today than at any other time in human history? Some human rights organizations estimate that as many as twenty million people worldwide are in bondage, and an alarming number of slaves are children. Spiritually speaking, you were born into slavery, but now, if you have placed your faith in Jesus Christ, you have been set free in order to be a slave to God.

In Paul's day, one in four persons was a slave, and many of those slaves had converted to Christianity. Consider the before and after picture Paul painted for them and us. Before you were saved by grace, you were a slave to sin, but now that you have been saved by grace, you are a slave to God, or at least that is what you are supposed to be. Being a slave to sin is described as a bondage that leads to death. Whereas being a slave to God is described as a blessing that leads to eternal life. The question is not, "Are you a slave?" The question is, "Whose slave are you?"

An addiction could be defined as the compulsive physiological or psychological need for a specific substance or activity to the point that it interferes with your relationships to other people, work, family, friends, and God. The addiction could be to something that is harmful or to something that is not necessarily harmful, but becomes harmful because of the unhealthy control it has on your life. A person who has become addicted to any substance or activity—whether cocaine, alcohol, prescription drugs, tobacco, caffeine, food, sex, or too much television—has become a slave to that substance or activity.

And here is Paul's point: You are a slave to God and therefore ought not to be a slave to anything else. Through grace, you have been set free from all addictions. Live in that freedom and become a slave to righteousness. "For the wages of sin is death, but the gift of God is eternal life in Christ Jesus our Lord" (v. 23).

DAILY HEALTH TIP

Joining a support group can be a healthy way to help overcome an addiction. Support groups let you know you are not alone and that you are not the only person struggling with your addiction. Support groups also make you accountable to other people. Find a Christ-centered, church-based support group and get involved. Trust Christ to transform your life.

QUESTIONS FOR REFLECTION

1. How would you describe the difference between being a slave to sin which leads to death and a slave to righteousness which leads to life? Whose slave are you?

2. How is an addict a slave to his or her addiction?

3. If a person has been set free through faith in Jesus Christ, why is it so easy to fall back into harmful addictions?

PRAYER FOR TODAY

Lord, my allegiance is to you. I pray that you would help me to overcome my dependence on anything other than your love and grace. Help me to rest contentedly in the good gifts that you provide. In the name of Jesus I pray. Amen.

DAY 3

1 CORINTHIANS 6:12–20

If we are not careful, we have a tendency to swerve into one of two ditches in trying to live the Christian way. One ditch is legalism. The legalist values keeping a list of rules and regulations. It causes us to think we are more spiritual than others when we are faithful to our list of rules in ways others are not. The other ditch, and just as dangerous, is license. License is the attitude that it really doesn't matter how I live my life since I am saved by grace. As long as I believe in Jesus, how I live my life is of little consequence. How do we stay in the lane and not swerve into either ditch?

Since we are saved by grace and not by the law, there is a temptation to think "everything is permissible for me" (v. 12). Practically, however, "not everything is beneficial" (v. 12). There may not be a specific amount of time that means you've watched too much TV, but watching twenty hours every day is not beneficial for you spiritually, physically, relationally, or emotionally. Technically, you may be able to justify many things, but practically, it's better to have the attitude that "I will not be mastered by anything" (v. 12) other than the Holy Spirit.

Some of the habits you have may seem harmless, but do they add value to your life? Do they make you a better father, mother, husband, wife, son, or daughter? Do they help your spiritual growth? If not, consider eliminating them, not because you have to, but because you desire to live a better, more abundant, total quality life.

Our natural impulses are temporary; we were created for more than satisfying our natural desires (vv. 13–17). Sacrificing what we temporarily desire for the sake of God has eternal value. Paul's advice was that we stay as far away from immorality as we possibly can. For all those other things that are permissible but not beneficial, Paul exhorted that our bodies are the dwelling place of the Holy Spirit, "Therefore honor God with your body" (v. 20).

DAILY HEALTH TIP

If you have any kind of addiction, talk to a professional. This could be a counselor or a minister. Talking to someone will shed light on your thought process and the circumstances that may trigger your addictive behavior. When you talk to a professional, make sure they have a Christian worldview and that you are completely honest with him or her. Failing to do both could do more harm than good.

QUESTIONS FOR REFLECTION

1. What are some habits you have justified because they are not really wrong even though they are not beneficial? Are you willing to let go of that habit in order to grow closer to God? Why or why not?

2. How, and in what ways, can you begin to "honor God with your body" (v. 20)?

PRAYER FOR TODAY

Dear God, I ask that you show me those things in my life that may be permissible but are not beneficial. Grant me the strength to give up those temporary impulses for eternal values. I thank you for your Holy Spirit that dwells within me. In Jesus' name I pray. Amen.

DAY 4

1 CORINTHIANS 8:1–13

The Christians living in Corinth could buy meat in the marketplace, where the meat was lower quality and higher priced, or at the local pagan temple, where the meat was higher quality and lower priced. The origin of the temple meat was well-known—it came from worshipers' offerings to a pagan god. The origin of the marketplace meat was often not known—it may have come from the temple or some other source.

As a result, Christians who consumed meat were faced with a dilemma: Should they shop for the best meat at a pagan temple or eat meat that could be associated with pagan worship? When they were guests in someone else's home and served meat that had been offered to idols, should they eat it?

Paul could have told the Corinthian believers to not worry about it and eat whatever they wanted whenever they wanted. But had he done this, he would have steered them into the ditch of license. Or, Paul could have advised them to avoid eating the meat under any condition. But had he done that, he would be steering them into the ditch of legalism.

Instead, Paul's advice to the Corinthian believers, as well as to us when we face those gray areas of not so right and not so wrong, was to exercise liberty with responsibility.

As a mature Christian, you may have discovered freedom, but you also have the responsibility to curb your liberty if it is going to harm a younger or more immature believer. Paul wrote, "Be careful, however, that the exercise of your freedom does not become a stumbling block to the weak" (v. 9). Furthermore, you should be willing to forsake, or cease to participate in that activity, even though you know it is not wrong, for the sake of the other, weaker person (v. 13).

When the Bible is clear, stand firm and don't compromise. But when the Bible is silent and there are differences of opinion among believers, be willing to curb your liberty for the sake of unity and maturity.

DAILY HEALTH TIP

Replace the time you might have spent participating in a questionable activity by volunteering that time to serve others. If you know that on a certain night of the week you will be tempted to do something you've chosen not to do, find a ministry organization that you can serve during that time instead.

QUESTIONS FOR REFLECTION

1. What are some issues believers face today about right and wrong that is similar to the issue in Paul's day about meat offered to idols? How do you usually handle a situation where believers see an issue or activity differently?

2. Why do you think Paul admonished those more mature in faith to compromise or refrain from certain activities for the sake of those weaker in faith?

PRAYER FOR TODAY

Lord, thank you for the simplicity and practicality of your Word. I pray you will help me see where I should give up my liberty for the sake of unity and maturity. God, help me to have the desire to give up things that are not wrong for the sake of you and others. In the wonderful name of Jesus I pray. Amen.

DAY 5

EPHESIANS 5:3–20

Paul made a list of things that should be avoided by a disciple of Jesus Christ. Some of the things are obvious, like sexual immorality and greed, but others are not so obvious, like "obscenity, foolish talk or coarse joking" (v. 4). When it comes to harmful substances, we usually think of things we put into our bodies, but here Paul mentions harmful substances that come out of our bodies through our speech. What goes in usually does come out. Jesus put it this way: "What goes into a man's mouth does not make him 'unclean,' but what comes out his mouth, that is what makes him 'unclean'" (Matt. 15:11).

Paul said that while you once were unclean, you are no longer to be that way because you have been brought from darkness to light (Eph. 5:8–11). "Live as children of light" (v. 8) and have nothing to do "with the fruitless deeds of darkness" (v. 11). As we have looked at the writings of Paul this week, a common theme has been that, though we were once unclean, we have been set free, so we ought to live like we have been set free.

This section closes with an admonition to be careful how we live because we represent Jesus Christ. As such, we shouldn't "get drunk on wine, which leads to debauchery. Instead be filled with the Spirit" (v. 18). Drunkenness is but one example. Whatever our addiction, we are to get rid of it and give ourselves instead to the control of the Holy Spirit. Lift other people up, encourage them in their journey of faith and "always [give] thanks to God the Father for everything, in the name of our Lord Jesus Christ" (v. 20).

DAILY HEALTH TIP

One of the most powerful weapons you have to fight addiction and return to a life of quality health is prayer. Prayer reminds you who is really in control, and it is through prayer you receive power to overcome. As you seek to be free of harmful substances and behaviors, don't forget to pray.

QUESTIONS FOR REFLECTION

1. What is the one thing you remember the most about your study this week? Why do you think that is the one thing that stands out?

2. What do you think is the relationship between the harmful substances people put in their bodies and the harmful statements that come out of their mouths?

3. What steps can you take today to surrender control of your life to the Holy Spirit?

PRAYER FOR TODAY

Lord, thank you for your convicting power and forgiving spirit. Thank you for the hope I have in Jesus and the help I have from the Holy Spirit. In Jesus' name I pray. Amen.

WEEK 6

HAVE REGULAR CHECK-UPS

RECOMMENDED READING

It's not fun getting older, but as you age, there are common-sense things you can do to gain and maintain total quality health. You know what those things are—exercise more, eat less, drink water, and get adequate rest. The only thing standing between you and better health is your determination and resolve to make changes in your life. However, some health problems are more significant and require professional medical treatment and oversight.

Many people hate going to the doctor. I am now at the age where I have to see my doctor at least once a year. Going to the doctor is not my favorite thing to do, but I am convinced that one of the best things a person can do to achieve total quality health is building a good relationship with their primary care doctor and visiting that doctor for check-ups on a regular basis.

Maintaining quality health by having regular check-ups is the topic for this week. These Bible studies will keep the topic of sickness, doctors, and healings in our minds, and the daily health tips will center on how to choose a primary care physician.

DAY 1

LUKE 1:1–4; ACTS 1:1–5; COLOSSIANS 4:14

I have always found it interesting that God chose a medical doctor to write two of the books in the New Testament. Luke, a physician, wrote the books of Luke and Acts in the Bible. A good medical doctor pays attention to details, and Luke made it clear at the beginning of both Luke and Acts that he was going to pay attention to details. But what else do we know about Dr. Luke?

More than likely, Luke was from Antioch. Not much is known about his life, and he is only referred to by name three times in the New Testament. It is obvious from his writings that he knew Theophilus, a wealthy government official. A common practice in that day was for wealthy slave owners to educate capable slaves as physicians and then grant them their freedom. There is some evidence that Luke was a common slave name, and some scholars have speculated that Luke was born as a slave in Theophilus's household, trained as a physician, and then granted freedom.

From the New Testament, we know that Luke traveled with Paul on some of his missionary journeys and was with Paul during his imprisonment in Caesarea. Luke was obviously a man of integrity and humility. His writings make up over one-fourth of the New Testament, but he never mentioned himself by name. His writings, especially his gospel, show that he was passionate about helping the poor, sick, and outcast. Luke truly had a physician's heart.

If you do not have a primary care physician, you need to find one. As you look for a doctor, look for someone who has the same characteristics as Dr. Luke. He was a man of faith, loyalty, humility, integrity, and compassion; he paid attention to details.

DAILY HEALTH TIP

When choosing a primary care doctor, the most important thing you can do is your homework. Make sure to get referrals from your family and friends, check the doctor's credentials and insurance coverage, and most importantly, ask lots of questions.

QUESTIONS FOR REFLECTION

1. What do you think are the most important characteristics of a doctor?

2. Why do you think some people hate going to the doctor? When was the last time you went to the doctor?

PRAYER FOR TODAY

Lord, thank you for choosing a man like Luke to write parts of the New Testament and for his example of faith, loyalty, integrity, and humility. Thank you, Father, for giving men and women today the capability of learning and practicing medicine. Please guide me in my choice of physicians and guide them in providing care for me. In Jesus' name I pray. Amen.

DAY 2

MATTHEW 9:9–13

In ancient Rome, individuals could purchase the rights to collect taxes from territories that had been conquered. Of the taxes collected, they would owe a certain amount to Rome, then pocket the rest. So, a tax collector could make as much money as he could extract from the people, completely protected by the government. In order to get such a job, Matthew must have already been a wealthy businessman; and the only reason to become a tax collector was to become even wealthier.

To a Jewish person in the first century, the only thing worse than a tax collector would have been a Jewish tax collector. They were considered traitors. The Jewish Talmud (an ancient commentary on the Old Testament) taught that it was righteous to lie and deceive a tax collector because it was what a professional extortionist deserved. Tax collectors were the lowest of the low. After Jesus reached out to Matthew, the tax collector invited Jesus to his house for dinner. Matthew's house was probably large enough to host a hundred or more guests, so this banquet probably included dozens more "tax collectors and 'sinners'" (v. 10) as guests. Jesus was keeping bad company, and the Pharisees later told him so. Jesus responded to the Pharisees, "It is not the healthy who need a doctor, but the sick. . . . For I have not come to call the righteous, but sinners" (vv. 12–13).

Jesus is the Great Physician. As his followers, we have the prescription that cures the loneliness, depression, and anxiety of lost people. We have the hope that the world needs. It is not the people who consider themselves healthy who will benefit from this cure; rather, it is those who recognize themselves as spiritually sick who can gain from the hope Jesus offers. It is time for all of us to become medical missionaries, reaching out to the sick and offering the mercy and grace of God.

DAILY HEALTH TIP

Once you have done your homework and chosen a doctor, schedule an appointment to get a complete physical examination. At the end of the examination, ask your doctor, "What do I need to do to improve my health?" Then, make a commitment to follow your doctor's advice.

QUESTIONS FOR REFLECTION

1. What do you think Jesus meant when he said, "It is not the healthy who need a doctor, but the sick" (v. 12)? How would you explain what he meant to someone else?

2. What implications does Jesus' statement have on how and to whom you reach out with the hope of Christ?

PRAYER FOR TODAY

Heavenly Father, I was spiritually sick and you healed me. What you did for me you can do for others. Help me to reach out to the sick, poor, and those who have no hope. Break my heart and fill me with compassion for the lost. In Jesus' name I pray. Amen.

DAY 3

JAMES 5:13–20

Occasionally, medical journals will publish articles about the effects of prayer on the healing process. Some studies seem to show that patients who pray have a quicker recovery from sickness and surgery. Often, the explanation given for the data is that people who pray and have others praying for them experience a greater sense of hope and support from their family and friends. The conclusions drawn typically leave little space for believing that prayer works because God answers prayer.

The word *trouble* in today's reading (v. 13) refers to hardship or distress. When such hardships come, our first response should be to pray. If, on the other hand, you are not suffering at the moment, you should "sing songs of praise" (v. 13). Every day—at every moment—you have a reason to either pray or praise.

James admonishes that if anyone is sick, they "should call the elders of the church to pray over him and anoint him with oil in the name of the Lord" (v. 14). Some of the most precious times I have had with my church family have been gathered around someone who is sick, praying for them, laying hands on them, and anointing them with oil. Miraculous healings can occur through such times. And even when God chooses not to heal, congregations grow closer through laying someone's sickness at God's feet. This is another kind of miracle.

Perhaps you know someone like the young mother who was told she had cancer. Her church fasted and prayed with her. And when she had her follow-up exam to determine the severity of the cancer, it was gone without a trace! While such dramatic results may not be everyday occurrences, God does still heal and forgive when we pray. "The prayer of a righteous man is powerful and effective" (v. 16). Go to your doctor; follow his or her advice; take your medicine; have that surgery. But through it all, don't forget to pray.

DAILY HEALTH TIP

The best time to choose a doctor is now, before you need one. When you are sick or in the middle of an emergency, you will not have the time to check referrals and do your homework. If you do not already have a doctor, begin the process of choosing one today. You will not be sorry.

QUESTIONS FOR REFLECTION

1. Do you believe God still heals? Why or why not? Do you know someone who experienced a miraculous healing?

2. Why do you think prayer works in helping people who are sick or recovering from a sickness? Do you believe in the power of prayer? Why or why not?

PRAYER FOR TODAY

Dear Jesus, you are the Great Physician, and I thank you for the privilege to bring my needs and concerns for friends, family, and myself to you. I trust in you to provide whatever kind of healing is most needed in the lives of those I love. I believe the prayer of faith makes me whole. In your almighty name I pray. Amen.

DAY 4

MARK 1:29–45

The Gospels were not intended to be a detailed (or even a chronological) biography of Jesus' life. The Gospels focus primarily on a three-year period of time, and the most space is dedicated to the last week of Jesus' life. But the glimpse these books give us of Jesus' ministry is meant to be a summary of the kinds of things he did and taught as he was inaugurating his kingdom, and the story we have is more than adequate. In fact, John said it would be impossible to write down everything that Jesus did (see John 20:30–31).

The day Mark described in today's passage started with Jesus traveling to Capernaum on the Sabbath and delivering a man from demon possession (see Mark 1:21–28). After leaving the synagogue, Jesus went to Peter's home and healed Peter's mother-in-law from a fever (vv. 29–31). That evening, "the whole town gathered at the door, and Jesus healed many who had various diseases" (vv. 33–34). Mark 1 ends with Jesus healing a man of leprosy (vv. 40–45).

Jesus said he "came to seek and to save what was lost" (Luke 19:10). The word *save* means "to be made whole again." So, Jesus came to make people whole—not only spiritually whole, but emotionally and physically whole as well. When Jesus heals a person, he makes that person whole and gives a glimpse into what life in his kingdom will be like. Our ultimate healing will come in the next life when we will live forever. But I am so thankful that, in this life, Jesus gives us a glimpse into heaven by healing us and making us whole again.

DAILY HEALTH TIP

In choosing a doctor, consider personal factors. Are you looking for a male or female doctor? It is vital that you feel comfortable with your doctor. You want a doctor who is kind, compassionate, and who will patiently listen to all your concerns and questions. Finally, take time to learn about the doctor's support staff. Chances are, when you call the office, those are the people who will answer your call.

QUESTIONS FOR REFLECTION

1. Have you ever imagined what it would have been like to have been an eyewitness to Jesus' life and ministry? If so, what are some of the things you imagined?

2. In what ways does being saved by Jesus mean to be made whole again? What areas of your life has Jesus made whole? What areas of your life need to be made whole?

PRAYER FOR TODAY

Dear God, I claim your sanctifying power to make me whole. Use me to bring your healing into someone else's life this week. In Jesus' name I pray these things. Amen.

DAY 5

Revelation 21:1–27

Our bodies are God's temple, so we need to do all we can to live a healthy life. In order to maintain total quality health, we need to eat right, exercise regularly, get adequate rest, reduce our stress levels, avoid harmful substances, and have regular check-ups. Ultimately, our bodies will deteriorate. However, by staying in the best shape possible, we make our lives more comfortable, enjoyable, and productive. The good news is that in the next life, for all eternity, we will be in perfect health.

In today's passage, John describes what the new heaven and new earth will look like. Actually, John only describes one city, the New Jerusalem. It's a beautiful picture. Our eternal home is far greater, far more magnificent than mere words can describe. Read the chapter slowly, multiple times. Try to picture what John is describing.

While all of Revelation 21 is important and beautiful, I want to focus on verse 4: "He will wipe every tear from their eyes. There will be no more death or mourning or crying or pain, for the old order of things has passed away."

Imagine that! In heaven, there will be no more death, mourning, or crying. I think it is safe to assume that among other things this means that in heaven there will be no more sickness, cancer, heart attacks, diabetes, obesity, colds, allergies, or headaches—no more sickness of any kind.

Why will these things be absent? Because on the new earth, "no longer will there be any curse" (22:3). Because of sin, this entire universe has been cursed (see Gen. 3). Once Jesus returns, the curse will be destroyed, along with sickness and death.

"Behold, I am coming soon! Blessed is he who keeps the words of the prophecy in this book" (Rev. 22:7).

"Amen. Come, Lord Jesus" (22:20).

DAILY HEALTH TIP

In choosing a doctor, make sure the doctor practices relatively close to where you live and that he or she has admitting privileges at your preferred hospital. You do not want to drive long distances for an appointment, and if you ever do need to be hospitalized, you need to be able to go to the hospital of your choice.

QUESTIONS FOR REFLECTION

1. If in the end everyone dies, even those who have been healed, why does it matter so much that we take care of our bodies?

2. What sickness are you or someone close to you dealing with today? What does it mean to you to know that in the next life there will be no sickness? How does believing that truth help you deal with your present circumstance?

PRAYER FOR TODAY

Heavenly Father, I am overwhelmed by your love for me and by your promise that I will spend eternity with you in a place that is beyond description. Set me apart to love and serve you all the days of my life. Preserve me in good health so that I can bring honor and glory to you. In the name of Jesus I pray. Amen.